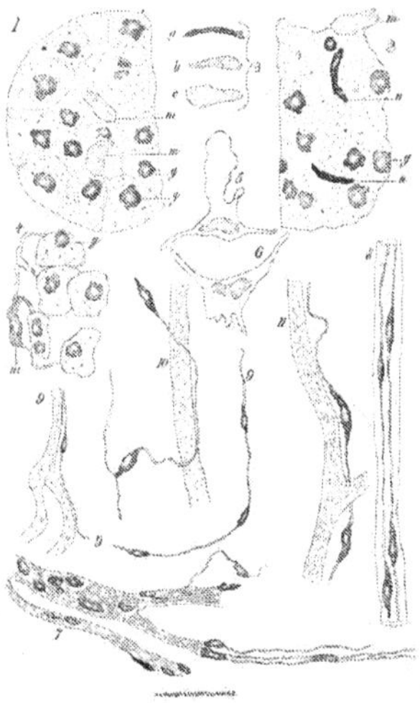

The Cleveland Medical Gazette

Vol. 1, No. 5, March 1886

A. R. Baker, S. W. Kelley, and Others

Originally Published in

1886

Contents

DESCRIPTION OF PLATE.

Powers used. Figs. 7 and 9, Gundlach's objective, III, ocular III, magn. about 175 diam. All the rest Gundlach's objective V, ocular III, magn. about 500 diam.

Fig. 1. Part of alveolus, submaxillary cat, compressed Carmine.

m. Nuclei of memb. propr.

g. Nuclei of gland cells.

Fig. 2. Part of alveolus submaxillary cat; membr. propr. torn Carmine.

n. Nuclei of membr. prop. either rolled up or seen edgewise.

m. Similar nucleus flattened out.

Fig. 3. Nucleus of membr. propr.

a. Viewed edgewise.

c. Viewed from surface.

b. Viewed in position between both.

Fig. 4. Group of gland cells with nucleus and portion of membr. propr. resembling a connective tissue corpuscle with processes.

Figs. 5 and 6. Fragments of membrana propria with nuclei. Cat.

Fig. 7. Nerve trunk with branches, accompanying a small duct. Carmine. In the main trunk the individual fibrils cannot be distinguished. Aniline blue might have made them distinct.

Fig 8. Small nerve trunk containing two naked fibrils in sheath. Aniline blue.

Fig. 9. Single naked nerve fibril found passing on to an alveolus. It seemed to pass on to the capillary figured but a small break, where the fibre might have been torn, or where from the underlying cells it could not be distinguished—allows doubt if the fibre seen along-side of the capillary is the continuation of the fibre. Carmine and aniline blue.

Figs. 10 and 11. Capillaries with nerve fibrils accompanying the same. Carmine and aniline blue.

THE

Cleveland Medical Gazette

THE Cleveland Medical Gazette

VOL. I. - MARCH, 1886. - No. 5.

ORIGINAL ARTICLES.

TWO DISPUTED POINTS IN THE HISTOLOGY OF THE SUBMAXILLARY GLAND. MEMBRANA PROPRIA—NERVE-ENDINGS (WITH PLATE.)[1]

BY CHR. SIHLER, M. D., PH. D., CLEVELAND, OHIO. Formerly Fellow of the Johns Hopkins University.

The submaxillary gland is of importance not only for its own sake, but because its anatomical connections and situation are such that it can be subjected to physiological experiment, and a number of important results have been reached which I may discuss at some future time.

1. Read before the Cuyahoga County Medical Society, January 7, 1886.

The results of my work are not only contradictory to the authorities in histology, but also do not harmonize with the requirements of prevailing physiological theories. Bringing this before you does not mean that I ask you to accept either facts or conclusions. I am fully aware of the difficulty of such work, the doubtfulness of the facts and the liability to error in the conclusion. But it is just possible that some of the younger members may fare as I did—have not all their time occupied by practice—and if I enlist the interest of any in this most important region I shall feel happy.

A number of years have passed since I undertook this question, and the work on the nerve-endings on muscle, which I had the pleasure to communicate to this society a few months ago, was undertaken more as a study, to make myself familiar with analogous structures, than that I expected to find anything new.

METHOD.

In the investigations on the nerve-endings I used the submaxillary of the half-grown cat, the calf, the ox and the puppy. The method followed was in the main that of Beale. In the case of the cat I injected the whole animal from the aorta with Turnbull's blue, dissected out the gland, duct, and the nerves entering it. After breaking up the gland into pieces by aid of a needle, from the size of a bean to a pea, I placed it in a dish with a light cover, containing Beale's carmine (carmine dissolved in ammonia and glycerine). I am in the habit of using a stronger solution than Beale's. I suspect that the carmine I used in some of these stainings was adulterated with eosin, and that possibly this may have been of advantage. In some of my stainings I used a fluid prepared from cochineal; used ammonia in dissolving the coloring matter, and then added carmine besides. It is of the utmost importance to have no excess of ammonia present, otherwise the staining will be slow and imperfect. I have been staining with this method for years, yet I cannot say why the results differ so much. Some time ago I stained a frog for the nerve-endings in muscle and obtained the most beautiful results, but in the number of stainings I have made since (trying to follow the same method) I have not been by far as successful as then. In breaking up the gland I do not always separate all the pieces, but try to remove the connective tissue holding together the small lobules with the dull end of a needle, and then throw the coherent mass into the stain. In this way I procured a very perfectly injected and beautifully stained submaxillary of a half-grown cat, from which I made a number of valuable specimens. The material may remain in the staining fluid for weeks, and may be examined every two or three days to note how the staining is advancing. When the masses stained are large, or the whole gland is subjected to staining, of course the outer parts are more deeply stained than the inner ones, but it is at times convenient to have material of different depths of staining. After the process has continued long enough—the nuclei at least should be very distinctly colored—the material is transferred into a fluid containing glycerine five parts, water and alcohol each two parts, acetic acid one part. Here it may remain about twenty-four hours, and finally it is to be preserved in a similar mixture containing but a trace of acetic acid. I hold acetic acid of varying strength diluted with glycerine in high esteem in such investigation. It does two things, removes the superfluous stain and softens and clears up the connective tissue. Thus treated, the material is ready for examination.

The tissues thus prepared may be hardened in alcohol and sections cut, but this will not aid much in the investigation of the questions that interest us. For this purpose teasing and compression with the cover glass are mainly to be relied upon. It is to be commended to isolate one of the little lobules the gland is composed of, because thus we certainly have ready for examination all the elements making up the gland. The little root which connects the lobule with the rest of the gland will consist of the duct, vessel and nerves supplying the lobule. Such a lobule is broken up with needles and by compression between slides. All these manipulations are to be carried on in glycerine. When the fragments are small enough they are examined with lower powers. The ducts in well injected specimens can be recognized by the rich supply of vessels, the nerve-trunks by the arrangement of the nuclei.

After examining larger fragments with lower powers, smaller ones are selected, subjected to pressure with cover glass, and examined with higher powers. By compression with cover glass, pushing from side to side, one can isolate almost any structure. One can also then make sure whether a fine fibre is really in connection with any other structure, or only lying above or beneath the same.

The staining with the carmine will generally not attack the fine nerve fibres. To show these up I have used aniline blue dissolved in water. By these means I have brought out very plainly the nerve fibres, in nerve trunks, of considerable size, as well as those along vessels. I took the material prepared as described, broke up a little piece in fragments of the size of mustard seeds, and left them twelve hours in the blue fluid in a watch glass. Glycerine, if necessary, slightly acidulated, will remove the superfluous stain. I was very much pleased with the action of the aniline blue.

Notwithstanding its physiological importance there is among the authorities as yet no uniformity of opinion on the histology of this gland, save that it belongs to the racemose glands, and is made up of epithelial cells.

The question whether there is present a special membrana propria, enveloping the glandular epithelium, as Pflüger teaches, or a network of partly coalesced connective tissue cells, as Kölliker supposes, may not seem very important, but certainly such points must be cleared up before such questions as to how the nerves end can satisfactorily be answered.

This question, the importance of which will be admitted by all, is also a disputed one. In Stricker's handbook Pflüger has, in the article on the submaxillary gland, given a detailed account of the mode of nerve-ending in this gland. According to his investigations it is of various kinds.

(1.) The medullary fibre approaches an alveolus penetrates this membrane, the axis cylinder breaks up into innumerable fine fibres, and these pass into the body of the gland cell. (2) Or the nerve passes into a pale cell provided with numerous processes, which in their turn form connections with the secreting cells.

These results of Pflüger have, however, not been accepted by all investigators. Thus Kölliker says on this question:

"The investigations on the nerve-endings in the salivary glands are evidently far from being concluded, nevertheless so much can be gathered from the work done that the nerve fibres are in more intimate relations with the glandular elements than has been surmised heretofore. What these relations may be I cannot say, for notwithstanding a very careful investigation of this gland it has not been possible for me to reach views definite and not open to doubt, although frequently enough I have seen fibres and threads of various kinds apparently come in contact with salivary cells. Further, regarding the drawings and descriptions of Pflüger, I must confess, having at the same time nothing but the highest esteem of this investigator, as well as of the care and accuracy he employed in this question, that these do not seem altogether convincing to me."

MEMBRANA PROPRIA.

I find that the gland cells are enclosed by a membrane (agreeing altogether with Pflüger) which I look upon as decidedly homogeneous (histologically speaking, of course), not showing any structure; by no means being merely a reticulum of connective tissue corpuscles, as Kölliker suggests.

Further: This membrane is provided with nuclei of an oval form (generally), reminding me of the nuclei supplying the nerve sheaths.

Finally: This membrana propria sends out from the alveolar walls, processes, ensheathing—how complete I cannot say—the gland cells. I cannot otherwise explain the glistening lines, which we see in examining sections VI extending from the alveolar wall between the cells, resembling altogether the sections of the alveolar walls. To investigate this matter more accurately, I have stained sections with carmine, also with log-wood, and have found that the alveolar wall and these lines stain the same way. Further breaking up such a section by manipulation with cover-glass, one can obtain fragments of these processes, thus demonstrating that these lines are not merely optical illusions.

The nuclei of this membrana propria are situated on its inner surface and could be distinguished in the gland of the cat, mentioned above, not only by their more oval, oblong or elliptical form, from the more roundish nuclei of the gland cells, but just as plainly by the lighter red or pinkish staining which they take on the nuclei of the gland cells being stained a deeper red.

Compressing very small fragments of gland-substance (always of course in glycerine), by means of the cover-glass, beating and pushing it from side to side, thus bursting the alveolus and tearing the membrane and isolating it from the contained gland cells, one can prepare for examination greater or smaller pieces of this membrane. There are by such means obtainable fragments with all sorts of processes and fringes, short and long, many and few, which undoubtedly may remind one of "connective tissue cells." (See fig. 4.) More convincing than these are membraneous pieces, which may be obtained of various sizes. (See figs. 5, 6.) I have a drawing of such a fragment, which, if enlarged as figs. 1 and 2, would cover over one-quarter of the page, and to which a number of nuclei, more than six, are attached. As a rule, this membrane will, by the manipulations with the cover-glass, not be spread out, but rather folded up, huddled together inclosing some of the gland cells, forming an indescribable nest.

I do not know if it will be necessary to mention in this connection that I consider these nuclei identical with the half-moon cells of Gianuzzi, and cannot help expressing my surprise at the physiological importance assigned to them; for they have been considered playing the role of mother cells, giving origin to glandular epithelium formed to take the place of cells used up in the process of secretion. The dark staining, which in section they seem to assume as well as the semilunar form, will be discussed later. Of course I look upon these nuclei as belonging to flat epithelial cells, as we find them lining nerve sheaths, and serous membranes, and consider them of the same physiological importance as the nuclei of such endothelial cells. A similar ensheathing membrane, or membrana propria, I find in the ducts; but here I have not been able to distinguish processes passing in between the cells. If present they must be exceedingly delicate, for it is not difficult to press out groups of cells from the ducts so that empty pieces (short ones of course) of such can be examined.

While the membrana propria of the ducts can be separated rather easily from the inclosed cells, it is different from the surrounding network of capillaries. It seems impossible to remove the capillaries from the duct-walls; while, in the gland-structure proper, among the alveoli, the separation of the capillary from an alveolus, can with little difficulty often be accomplished, so that a piece of capillary can be examined without any other structures lying above or beneath it.

BLOODVESSELS.

It was somewhat surprising to me, and not a little interesting, to find that the ducts have a decidedly richer blood supply than the gland substance proper, the meshes of the capillaries covering the ducts very closely indeed.

I will also call attention to the fact that, along the terminal portions of the ducts, no arteries or veins can be seen; and what is still more important, no free nerve-fibres can be discovered. Following the ducts outwards, as these attain larger dimensions, and especially where they give off side branches, we find arteries and veins accompanying them, and there will also be found alongside of them fine nerve-branches. So much is certain, that in that region, where arteries and veins are not to be seen, there are also no separate nerve twigs, and that here the union or coalescence of nerve and tissue which the nerves are to influence must have taken place. If one considers the fine meshes of the capillary network enveloping the ducts, and keeps in mind the abundance of nuclei belonging to the capillary, the membrana propria and the duct cells proper, he can imagine how difficult it must be to follow the course of the nerves through and among all these structures. That it has been impossible for me to separate capillary and membrana propria, has been mentioned.

NERVES.

If one were to ask the physiologist: What do you expect us to find in our anatomical investigations on the nerve-endings in the submaxillary gland, he would undoubtedly answer: "You will find an arrangement analogous, if not similar, to that in the striped muscle; the nerve-fibre will be seen to approach the alveolus, penetrate its covering, and the protoplasm of the nerve and the gland-cell will be found to come in contact, if not to coalesce." And that is what has been found by Pflüger.

It has been my endeavor for some time to find something similar to the descriptions of Pflüger, but so far in vain, although many an alveolus has been carefully examined, flattened out and slowly crushed, so that each nucleus could be diagnosed, but never have I found anything which would remind me of the drawings by Pflüger in Stricker's 'Histological Handbook.'

In this matter I reasoned thus: If there are any such structures as specialized nerve-endings present in the glandular elements, we might look for an analogy either to the striped muscle fibres or to the capillaries, in both of which nerve-endings are known to be present. In the former case we have the so-called end-plate—the nerve fibre ends in a multi-nucleated mass—but as the muscle fibre, standing for a number of cells, is so different a structure from the gland-cells, we might, with greater probability, expect some such arrangement as we see on the capillaries. Here we see fine fibrils, provided with nuclei, exceeding the fibres two to four times in thickness, entwining the capillary, thus coming in contact with each of the cells composing the capillary wall. In the (submaxillary) gland there are similar structures to be influenced; at least in the capillary as well as in the gland, we have cells lying side by side to be influenced by nerves—hence we might expect similar structures.

Although the books in general have very little to say about the nerve supply of the capillaries, yet it is a fact, and can well be demonstrated, *e. g.*, in the frog's muscle, that such is the arrangement. As a rule, the fibril cannot so readily be detected, but the nuclei belonging to it are not difficult to recognize. A still more convenient and instructive locality is the base of the frog's mouth, where everything is one plane, and where the nerve fibres can be followed to their ultimate ramifications.

Let us now see what evidence of nerve-endings we find in or on the alveoli of the gland, examining one, or more accurately, a part of one (the round eminence). We shall see what fig. 1 presents. We see there two sets of nuclei; one kind oval, longish, stained lighter than the rest, of a pink hue (fig. 1, *m*), and these a further examination will demonstrate to be the nuclei belonging to the membrana propria, which have also been described before. Besides these nuclei, fewer in number, there is another kind, making up the bulk of the nuclei, more rounded in form (fig. 1, *g*), and of a deep-red color, which, in their turn, will prove to be the nuclei of the gland-cells; and these two are the only elements or structures that I have been able to demonstrate in a glandular alveolus.

At one time I thought I had found in or on the alveoli the evidence of a network of fine nerves. Quite frequently one can observe longish, even spindle-shaped, often deeply stained, nuclei, which resemble very much those belonging to the fine nerve fibres. (Fig. 2, *n*, such nuclei are figured.) But so far, whenever I examined such a spindle-shaped nucleus more carefully,

I found that it proved to be one of the nuclei belonging to the membrana propria, already described, and the form, as well as its dark color, was due to the fact that it had been examined edgewise. If, by manipulation, such a nucleus was turned over and compressed to present a flat surface, it would have an oval outline and be of a light-red color. Fig. 3 (*a*, *b*, *c*), shows the same nucleus as it appeared when seen edgewise, when seen from the flat and when seen in a position midway between these. Thus is also to be explained the demilune: If the section would strike a nucleus so that it would be seen only edgewise—especially if the membrana propria has a chance to roll up slightly—we should then have a deeply stained body, somewhat half-moon-shaped, the demilunes of the books.

So far, nothing but the nuclei have been mentioned, and the observation might very appropriately be made, that there might exist some exceedingly fine and delicate nerve fibrils without nuclei. Such a system of structures would, of course, be almost impossible to demonstrate with any degree of certainty. I have not, of course, sufficient reason to deny such an arrangement, and would not consider it improbable if we had not, in the capillaries of the frog's muscle (and other structures) evidence certainly not in favor of such an assumption. The fine nerve fibrils supplying the capillaries are richly supplied with nuclei, although the cells which build up the walls of the capillary are by far more insignificant elements than the secreting cells of the gland. Certain it is that as yet there is no evidence of the existence of such fine non-nucleated fibrils, arranged either in the form of a network or a bundle of fine branches.

The examination of the alveoli not leading to any results as to nerve-endings—no structures being discovered there that might be called nervous—I attacked the problem from the other side. I took up the nerve trunks accompanying the ducts, and tried how far I could follow their divisions and branches, and can say that I have spent a great deal of time on this point. In speakings of the bloodvessels, the fact was mentioned that, where arteries and veins of any size run along-side of the duct, these are accompanied by nerve branches, *i. e.*, bundles of nerve fibres, inclosed in a sheath, and these—at least in the cat, the calf and the ox—are made up (excepting, possibly, the very large trunks) of fine nerve fibres. Thicker or medullary nerves I have not been able to discover, even in branches of considerable size, consisting of, say six or eight fibres, and giving off smaller twigs containing one to three fibres. Fig. 7 shows such a nerve-trunk with side branches; neither in the main stem nor in the offshoots are there any medullary nerves discoverable.

If this observation is correct, we see that what has to be traced further, is not the more easily recognized medullary fibre, but exceedingly fine fibrils carrying in certain intervals nuclei, the only distinguishing feature. It will be admitted also (first) that it must be a matter of considerable difficulty to follow such indifferent looking structures, as delicate fibres. And (secondly), one cannot expect to find medullary nerves approach the alveoli, penetrate the membrane, come in connection with the secretory cells, etc., etc, as has been done by Pflüger. If the question should be asked how far I have been able to follow these nerves, I should say: Small twigs consisting of one to three fine fibrils, enclosed in a sheath branch off from a trunk, not much larger, and apply themselves to the membrana propria of the duct; their sheaths in all probability coalescing with that membrane. Here they have been seen to apply themselves to some bloodvessel and are now lost out of sight, being hid by all the many structures mentioned above, the nuclei of membrane, capillary, duct cells, and the fibre cannot so readily be distinguished from the membrana propria of the duct upon which it rests. But I do not wish to be understood that because the nerves have been lost out of sight, along-side of vessels, that they have their "ending" there, inasmuch as the network of bloodvessels is such a close one that the nerves cannot but help coming in contact with them. Fig. 8 shows such a fine nerve-trunk. By the aid of aniline blue the fine fibrils have been made quite plain. Such fine fibrils can by the same means be demonstrated in much larger trunks, as shown in fig. 7, and it can be shown that even such large trunks consist of nothing but these fine fibrils.

I have also seen, exceptionally however, fine nerve twigs run into the alveoli directly, but the nerves here were of the same nature as the ones described going to the duct. Fig. 9 shows a fine fibril passing on to an alveolus and running probably on to a vessel; the nerve fibre resting upon gland cells, also stained, could not with absolute certainty be traced to the vessel. There is a small break shown in the drawing.

As intimated, especially if the cells of the duct are still *insitu*, it is impossible to follow the fine nerve-fibres any further. By pressing out the cells from the ducts, one can obtain portion of the duct, with the capillaries belonging to them, but they are short pieces, and the nerve fibril is not easily discoverable.

But there remains one fact to be mentioned, which may throw light on the question, as to how the nerves end and which in my opinion might and does clear up the difficulty.

Examining the capillaries supplying the gland alveoli, one is able to find nuclei, not belonging to the capillaries themselves. This statement can be made for two reasons. In the first place, the majority of these nuclei have not the form of the nuclei of the capillary, and in the second place these nuclei are situated on the outside of the capillary wall. Whoever has examined the capillaries of the frog's muscle knows that just such or the same nuclei belong to nerve-fibres, supplying the capillary wall. In the mammal of course these nuclei are smaller and not so conspicuous, nor can we procure pieces of capilliary of any length (the structures under examination here, not being in one plane.) Thus we cannot expect to have matters so plain here and easy of demonstration. After finding these nuclei, it was of course my desire to find if they were united by fibres. It must in this matter be kept in mind, that if there are such fibres present to which these nuclei belong, these may be expected to be in the most intimate relation with the capilliary wall, if one is to influence the other—and therefore not of ready and easy demonstration.

I have, however, succeeded in showing in a number of instances that such fibres exist. Figs. 10 and 11 show such a fibre uniting several nuclei. The shortness of these fragments makes a more perfect demonstration almost impossible.

If this observation is correct, we find on the capillaries the same (only finer) fibres provided with nuclei, which we have lost out of sight following the branching out of the nerves.

There is also some evidence of fine fibres in the membrana propria of the ducts, inasmuch as we find here nuclei along-side of the capillaries, these not being the nuclei of the membrane, but resembling altogether the nuclei of the nerve fibres.

Again, as stated above, I have not been able to find any such evidence of nerves in connection with the gland cells themselves. In case, however, such an arrangement or something similar existed, why should it have been impossible for me to find evidences of such as well here on the gland cells as on the capillaries; and should they not be more readily found in the gland than in the capillary, inasmuch as we have larger structures to deal with here in the gland.

The conclusion then regarding the nerve-endings to which my work has led me are these:

There were no special nerve-endings found in connection with the gland cells themselves. *We find, however, upon thecapillaries evidence of the same kind of fine nucleated fibrils, whichwe find to be present in the fine nerve twigs*, as far as we can follow them in their course towards their final distribution. To explain the action of nerves on the process of secretion we would have to assume either that the nerves accompanying the capillaries also influence the gland cells, or that the glands are stimulated to activity by some changes in the condition of the capillary wall furnishing a greater amount of oxygen and nutritive fluids.

The results are partly negative, partly positive. The latter I wish to emphasize, believing it worthy of attention, as it may throw light on the physiology of the capillary wall, which seems to be altogether too much neglected. The negative I have offered, knowing well enough that such negative results must be accepted as final with much hesitation.

To any one feeling inclined to undertake investigation on this gland, I would make a few suggestions:

(1) Make sections through gland hardened in bichromate of potash, or alcohol, and stain with staining fluids.

(2) Compare in material prepared as above described, the vascular supply of duct and gland substance proper.

(3) Compare gland and duct cells.

(4) Find the nuclei of the membrana propria and compare the same with the nuclei of the gland cells.

(5) See if you can examine the same nucleus from different sides. Do you think that the demilune of books and the nucleus of the membrana propria might be the same thing?

(6) Prepare pieces of the membrana propria covering the alveoli. What is your opinion—is there a membrane or only a reticulum of connective tissue cells?

(7) Prepare pieces of membrana propria of duct.

(8) Can you find the nuclei of the duct, and other nuclei on the exterior of the capillaries?

(9) Can you find pieces of capillaries belonging to the alveoli, and do you find any nuclei on them?

(10) Examine the wall of the duct in injected and uninjected material, both stained.

(11) Follow the bloodvessels—can you find nerves on the walls of arteries?

(12) Of what structure do you find the root of a little lobule to consist?

(13) How do the nerve trunks differ from the fibrous envelope holding together all these structures?

(14) Differentiate between the nuclei of the nerve fibres and the nuclei of the nerve sheath.

(15) Examine nerve branches of various thicknesses—what do you find the nature of the nerve fibres to be? Do not forget the aniline blue and try other staining fluids.

(16) Can you find evidence in the alveoli of other structures besides capillary, membrana propria and salivary cells?

(17) How far have you succeeded in following the fine nerve twigs?

(18) By all means try different methods, different tissue, and compare the results. See what you can discover by simply teasing material treated with Muller's fluid, and other stained and treated as I have described.

(19) Follow the course of the arteries, and note where the larger vessels pass into the capillaries.

A HISTORY OF MEDICINE.

BY JOHN BENNITT, M. D., Professor of Principles and Practice of Medicine in the Medical Department of the Western Reserve University, Cleveland, Ohio. [*Continued from page 103.*]

But the contributions to medicine of all his predecessors dwarf into insignificance when compared to those of Galen—who lived and wrote in the middle of the second century—and whose writings were ultimate authority, until they were attacked and publicly burned in the 16th century by the arch-quack Paracelsus. Galen, although born in Pergamus, in Mysia and living there, was called by the Emperors M. Aurelius, and L. Verus to attend them in the northeastern frontier of Italy, and was for a considerable period of time physician to the emperor, spending a considerable portion of the last half of his life at Rome. He died in Sicily in 201 aet 71 (?) There are ascribed to him 83 treatises on medicine about which there is no question as to their genuineness, 19 that are questionable, 45 undoubtedly spurious, 19 fragments, 15 commentaries on Hippocrates' works. Besides these, he wrote a great number of works (not all on medicine) whose titles only are preserved, so that altogether it is believed that the number of distinct treatises cannot have been less than 500. These were, on (1) Anatomy and Physiology, (2) Dietetics and Hygiene, (3) Pathology, (4) Semiology and Diagnosis, (5) Materia Medica and Pharmacy, (6) Therapeutics including Surgery, (7) Commentaries on Hippocrates, (8) Philosophical and Miscellaneous. Most of these works are still extant in Greek (in which they were originally written). They have been translated into many modern languages. His works on anatomy and physiology are most valuable. But it is not certain that he ever dissected human bodies. His knowledge he derived from dissecting apes, bears, goats, etc., and his knowledge of physiology from experiments on these animals. His pathology was speculative.

In diagnosis and prognosis he laid great stress upon the pulse, on which subject he may be considered as the first and greatest authority, for subsequent writers adopted his system without alteration. He placed great confidence in the doctrine of "critical days," which he believed to be influenced by the moon.

In materia medica he was not considered as good authority as Dioscorides. He was prone to making prescriptions containing many ingredients, some of which were entirely *inert.* He seems to have placed more faith in amulets than in medicine, and is supposed to be the author of the anodyne necklace, which was for a long time famous in England. He was an allopathist in his notions, *i. e.*, he believed that disease is something contrary to nature, and is to be overcome by that which is contrary to the disease itself. At the same time he taught that nature is to be preserved by that which has relations to nature, in accord. Hence his two indications, "Overcome Disease," "Sustain Nature."

Before this time, as already intimated, the medical profession was divided into several sects, who were always disputing with one another. After him, all these sects seem to have merged into his followers. The subsequent Greek and Roman medical writers were compilers from his writings, and being translated into Arabic, Galen's works became authority in the East as well as in Europe, and continued to be so for fourteen hundred years. In 1559, Dr. Geynes was cited before the college of physicians for impugning the infallibility of Galen. On his acknowledgment of his error and humble recantation, signed with his own hand, he was received into the college.

The great mass of Galen's *works*, together with modern improvements and researches, have now in great measure consigned them to neglect, but his *fame* can only perish with the science itself. As in the case of Hippocrates, his immeasurable superiority over his contemporaries seems to have acted as a check to all attempts at further improvement.

The first names of any renown that occur subsequent to Galen are those of Oribasius, Alexander of Tralles, Ætius and Paulus Egineta, who flourished between the fourth and seventh centuries. They were all jealous Galenists, and those of their writings which are still extant are, for the most part, compilations from the predecessors, especially from their great master, Galen.

The writings of Paulus seem to be the last of any written in the Greek language, which had been the language of medical science for more than a thousand years. At about this time the Arabian school was beginning to rise into notice. The earliest Arabian writers on medicine of whom we have any notice or certain account, is Ahrum, who was contemporary with Paulus. The most celebrated physicians of this school were Rhazes, (who flourished in the ninth century, and was the first to describe small-pox) and Avicenna who flourished early in the eleventh century, and whose 'Canon Medicina' may be regarded as a cyclopaedia of all that was known of medicine at that time (as well as collateral sciences). This was a compilation from Greek writers, whose writings had been translated into Arabic, (for Avicenna was not a Greek scholar himself). Avenzoar, and Averrhoes flourished in the twelfth century. The last was a celebrated philosopher as well as physician. The works of Hippocrates and Galen, which, together with the works of Aristotle, Plato and Euclid, were translated into Arabic in the ninth century, formed the basis of their medical knowledge; but the Arabian physicians did good service to medicine, introducing new articles from the East into European materia medica, as for example, rhubarb, cassia, senna, camphor, and in making known what may be termed the first elements of pharmaceutical chemistry, such as a knowledge of distillation, and of the means of obtaining various metallic oxides and salts.

Upon the decline of the Saracenic universities in Spain, which was about the time of the death of Averrhoes, the only medical knowledge that remained was to be found in Italy, where the School of Salerno acquired considerable celebrity, which it maintained for some time, till it was gradually eclipsed by the rising fame of other medical schools at Bologna—where Mondino or Mundinus de Leozza publicly dissected two human bodies in 1315.

Contemporary with Mondini, lived Gilbert, the first English writer on medicine who acquired any repute; and the next century gave birth to Linacre, who after studying at Oxford spent a considerable time at Bologna, Florence, Rome, Venice and Padua, and subsequently became the founder of the London College of Physicians. It was in this fifteenth century that the sect of chemical physicians arose, who claimed that all the phenomena of the living body could be explained by the same chemical laws as those that rule inorganic matters. Although the illustrations and proofs which they adduced were completely unsatisfactory, yet the tendency at the present time is in the same direction, since chemistry and physiology are better known.

This seems to be a period prolific of new diseases. In the thirteenth, fourteenth and fifteenth centuries we hear most of leprosy, and of the visitation of the plague in Europe. Whooping-cough and scurvy were never described by any writer anterior to the fifteenth century. Syphilis was first recognized in Italy in the fifteenth century, from which country it spread rapidly over the whole of Europe.

In the sixteenth century the study of human anatomy may be said to have been fairly established by the zeal and labors of Vesalius, and in this and the succeeding centuries we meet with the names of many physicians whose anatomical and physiological investigations tended either directly or indirectly to advance the science of medicine. This was the epoch of Eustachius, Fallopius, Asellius, Harvey, Rudbeck, Bartholini, Malpighi, Glisson, Sylvius, Willis, Bellini, etc., names preserved in anatomy.

Chemistry was now being separated from alchemy, and advancing to a science, and a combination formed between its principles and those of physiology, which gave rise to a new sect of chemical physicians, quite distinct from the sect represented two centuries before by Paracelsus. The chemical school was succeeded by the mathematical school, of which Borelli, Sauvages, Heill, Jurin, Mead and Freind were amongst the most celebrated. While at the same time the old Galenists were fast disappearing. To the rival sects of this period must be added the Vitalists, which originated with Von Helmont, and with some modifications was adopted by Stahl and Hoffman. The greatest physician of the seventeenth century was, however, Sydenham, who, though inclining to the chemical school, did not allow his speculative opinions regarding the nature of disease to interfere with a careful consideration of the indications for treatment, as derived from the symptoms, and from experience.

Boerhaave, a Dutch physician and philosopher, occupied special prominence in last part of the seventeenth and the early part of the eighteenth centuries. He engaged in the practice of medicine at Leyden in 1693, and became professor of theory and practice of medicine in the university of that city in 1701. He was erudite, exact, simple and eloquent, and hence as a lecturer very popular. He specially advocated simplicity in practice of medicine. Professor of botany was added to his duties in 1709. He wrote a treatise in 1703 (in Latin) advocating mechanical and chemical hypotheses in medicine. In 1708 his institutes of medicine extended his reputation; and in 1709 appeared his famous 'Aphorisms' on the diagnosis and cure of disease. In this was a well defined classification of diseases, including their causes, nature and treatment, which was adopted by his contemporaries. He was distinguished as a botanist and chemist. He published a description of plants at Leyden in 1710, and became professor of chemistry in 1718 in addition to his other duties. He made chemistry popular by presenting it in a clear and attractive style, in his lectures and in his 'Elements of Chemistry' (1724).

On account of his attack of gout he was constrained to give up the teaching of botany and chemistry in 1727. He was elected a Fellow of the Royal Society of London in 1730. His fame extended over the world. A Chinese mandarin hearing of his fame addressed a letter to Boerhaave, physician in Europe, which reached him in due time. His practice was lucrative, and he spent money freely in the interest of science and benevolence, yet such was his success that it is said that at his death (in 1738) he left an estate of nearly a million dollars.

Cullen, who was born in 1710 and died in 1790, was undoubtedly the greatest medical man of his age. It is especially interesting to read the biographies of such men as Cullen and of Hunter his contemporary, and of Jenner of the last half of the eighteenth century, and of John Brown the quack—though much quoted.

The present century may be considered as the epoch of physiological experiment and clinical observation. The efficient laborers of the last eighty years in the field of medicine have been so numerous that it would be impossible to notice at this time even those deemed most celebrated, while it would be invidious to attempt such a selection.

In this time our materia medica has received a large number of most important additions, amongst which may be noticed, morphia, quinia, strychnia, iodine and the iodides, bromides, cyanohydric acid, cod-liver oil, chloroform, chloral, nitrite, amyl and a long list of preparations from the vegetable kingdom and from the hydrocarbon series.

The physical diagnosis of disease has been facilitated to an extent far beyond what the most sanguine physician of the last century could have deemed possible, by the discovery and practical application of the stethoscope, the pleximeter, the speculum in various forms, the ophthalmoscope, the laryngoscope and the thermometer; while chemistry and the microscopy have been applied successfully to the investigation of the various excretions, and especially of the urine, bile, and in the study of digestion where the process could be observed in its various stages in the person of Alexis St. Martin.

But the field for the medical historian broadens immensely and can best be appreciated by study of a catalogue of medical books and periodicals of the present century.

CASE OF HYSTERICAL BLINDNESS.

BY D. B. SMITH, M. D. Professor of Diseases of the Eye and Ear in the Medical Department of Western Reserve University.

On the fourth day of June I was called to see Miss C. R., aged nineteen years, a clerk, who told me that she had gone to bed the night before perfectly well, and that when she awoke in the morning she found herself totally blind, and had remained so up to the time of my visit, about eleven o'clock. This blindness she said had come on without the least pain or bad feeling, and the eyes were not in the least degree uncomfortable, nor had they been during the morning. No cause on the part of the patient could be assigned for the attack, and nothing of the kind had ever happened to any member of the family before. The external examination gave not the slightest evidence of any disease of the eyeballs or lids. The conjunctiva was perfectly normal, as were also the cornea iris and pupil. The ophthalmoscope revealed a perfectly healthy retina and optic nerve and clear media. The tension of the eyeball was normal. There was not the least constitutional disturbance, if we except a marked nervousness caused by the fear that she would be permanently blind. The patient declared most positively that she could not see the lamp even when held close to the eyes. From the fact that the pupils were perfectly normal and moveable under the influence of light, and that the patient put out her hand to shake hands with me in a way that I felt she could not do if she did not see, I diagnosed a case of hysterical blindness. It was more than a simulated blindness, for all the anxiety and mental distress of actual blindness were present; and I am satisfied the patient was honest in her belief that she could not see. The ordinary remedies for hysteria were given and were taken faithfully and regularly, and although for several days she took large doses of the bromide, valerianate of ammonia, hyoscyamus, assafœtida, and kindred drugs, there was not the slightest improvement in her vision. These remedies were continued from the fourth to the fourteenth without any perceptible effect. After ten days I began to give her tonics instead, and although she took the elixir cinchona with dilute hydrochloric acid, tincture of nux vomica, quinine, iron oxid of zinc, and finally stimulants, there was no improvement and the patient said she remained in total darkness. This tonic course was continued up to the twenty-ninth, and had been followed out thoroughly for two full weeks without effect.

During the nearly four weeks treatment the patient said that when the eyes were shut she could discern the position of the lighted lamp, but when the eyes were open she could not see the lamp or the slightest object, or even tell daylight from darkness. At various intervals during this time her pastor visited her and offered her his most heartfelt sympathy. Her friends were becoming exceedingly anxious least the sight would never return, although I could assure them that there was not the least danger of permanent blindness. I became satisfied at this time that medication was not going to dispel this peculiar attack of hysteria and that it would need something besides medicine to produce such an impression upon her mind that she could overcome it, so I told her that I was going to do something the next day that would surely make her see before night, and that she should be of good cheer for her sight would return very soon. The next morning I went down about nine o'clock armed with my ophthalmoscope, my case of trial glasses and my Hearteloup's artificial leech. The patient seemed to be quite confident that she would soon see, and was very hopeful as to the result of what was to be done. I looked into the eyes with my ophthalmoscope, and then applied the cylinder of the artificial leech to the temples without scarifying and used considerable traction, first on one side and then on the other, having previously told her not to open the eyes until I told her to do so. In about half an hour I told her to open the eyes gradually so as not to let the light in too suddenly and then tell me what she could see. The instant she opened them she said I can see the light and the position of the window. I then told her to close the eyes again and I reapplied the cylinder and commenced the suction as before. By this time the temples had become red and so sensitive that she now complained of some pain when the cylinder was reapplied. After twenty minutes she was told to open the eyes again and she said she could see objects about the room distinctly. She was then tried with large letters but she said she could not see to read them, but could see the black objects. Told her glasses would help her and placed a No. 72 convex spherical glass before the eyes when she could see Jaeger No. 20, then told her she needed other glasses and replaced the No. 72. She now saw to read No. 16. I continued taking off and putting on this same No. 72, with good effect and whenever she came to a standstill in reading reapplied the cylinder with uniform benefit until finally after two hours constant work she could read Jaeger No. 1. During all this day she was able to see distinctly. The next day she was again unable to read but a short repetition of the same course brought her vision back again. There was no return of the blindness after that except occasionally for a short time at intervals of two or three days.

In the course of ten days all trace of the difficulty had passed by and since has never returned. This case was diagnosed as one of genuine hysteria and not one of simulating blindness or malingering, and is reported as the most marked case I have ever had illustrating the effect of hokus pokusing (to call it by a mild name) which produced such a strong mental impression that the patient lost sight of her own peculiar mental condition, and by which a perfect cure was effected.

To her the blindness was real, and her friends feel that a remarkable cure has been performed. Such a blindness can occur in any nervous hysterical patient, while simulated blindness usually occurs in those who wish to avoid service in the army or navy, or in the case of lazy young people who do not wish to study at school or college, and in those who have received a slight injury and wish to make it appear more serious for the sake of obtaining large damages, either from private individuals or corporations.

For its detection there are several methods which are usually sufficient to give us positive proof that the blindness is not real. Von Graefe placed a number eight or ten prism in front of the eye, with the base upwards, downwards or sidewise, and if strabismus is present before the removal of the prism there is binocular vision.

Juler places spectacles with an opaque glass in front of the good eye, when, if the patient can read, he must see with both eyes; or he places concave 20 before the good eye, when if the patient can read fine print he must see it with the other eye.

Juval places a ruler before the eye so as to cover part of the page to be read, when, if one eye is blind, not all the page can be read.

Mittendorf puts atropine in the good eye, when if the patient can read fine print he is not blind with the other eye.

Wells places a prism in front of the supposed blind eye, and notices whether the apis of vision of that eye changes when the prism is removed.

Bull bandages the good eye and places a prism in front of the other eye, and holds a lighted candle before the eye, and if the eye turns as the prism is turned, the eye is not blind.

The test with Snellens or other colored letters is also a good one. A word with alternate red and bluish green letters is painted on glass and placed in the window, and the patient is asked to read the letters. If a bluish green glass is held in front of the good eye, he will see only the green letters unless he can see with the other eye, for all but the red rays in the red letters are cut off in the transparency in the window, and the green glass cuts the red off, leaving those letters a perfect blank to the well eye.

Kugel places various colored glasses before each eye and then places an opaque glass in front of the sound eye, and a transparent glass of the same color before the other one, and if the patient sees the object, he is simulating blindness.

Herring has the patient look through a tube large enough to cover both eyes, and then suspends a small ball in front of the tube and drops small objects near this ball, and if the patient can tell whether the balls are dropped in front of or behind the suspended ball, he must see with both eyes.

Lawrence recommends the stereoscope for detecting binocular vision, and places in a covered stereoscope a picture each side of which is different, and yet such as to make a single picture when both sides are seen. A clock dial, for example, with figures in one side only or figures with complemental colors, such that with both eyes the object would appear differently colored from what it would when seen with either eye separately. The distance apart of two objects held up in front of both eyes can be readily told by the patient if he sees with both eyes, no matter how the objects are held with relation to each other. But if there is vision with one eye only, the patient can tell the distant apart with accuracy only when the objects are both held at the same distance from the eye, but not when one is held considerably in front of the other.

One who sees with one eye only always thinks he is nearer to the object than he really is when reaching out for that object. It is always more difficult for him to pour from a pitcher into a cup or glass if held a little distance below it, hence the blind in one eye usually place the nose of the pitcher in contact with the glass before pouring. The old parlor trick of placing two pins in the wall and putting a cent on them and directing the patient to stand across the room and then walk over to the cent and knock it off with the outstretched finger without hitting the pins, may be made use of as a test in simulated blindness, for with one eye the patient always falls short of the mark the first time the experiment is tried. The most simple method of detecting simulated blindness in one eye is by noticing the movement of the pupil under the influence of light. If an eye is blind, the light has little or no effect upon it when the other eye is closed. The pupil is usually dilated. It may be well to mention here that atropine dilatation is generally wider than that due to amaurosis, and also that a cone of light from a strong convex glass thrown upon the sound eye will contract the pupil of the blind eye if the dilatation is not due to atropine. Simulated blindness in both eyes is not likely to be seen, and then the condition of the pupil is of great value in detecting it, and is one of the best guides in connection with the ophthalmoscopic observation.

A CASE OF DOUBLE UTERUS AND VAGINA.

BY S. W. KELLEY, M. D., CLEVELAND, O.

Miss H. E., aged 20, American of Irish parentage: dark brunette, short in stature but apparently quite handsomely formed, and ruddy with health. She has never been sick in her life. Has menstruated normally since her fifteenth year, though scantily during the past year. She feared she had been injured a few days previously by the overturning of a chair upon which she was standing, as she had since felt pain and uneasiness in the lower pelvic and pubic region, for which she sought advice.

Upon examination I found no injury worthy of record, but the malformation here described. Cases of this anomaly have been recorded from time to time, being always of interest to the teratologist, occasionally requiring attention on account of interference with the marital relation or parturition, and being referred to in every discussion on superfœtation.

The external genitalia are well developed. No hymen, nor any remains of one. I have no reason to doubt her virginity. An inch within the introitus vaginæ the finger met a narrowing into which only its tip would pass. Searching to the left another smaller opening was discovered, the two being separated by a strong membrane. Returning to the right or larger passage, was able by careful dilatation for ten or fifteen minutes to insert three-fourths of the length of the index finger and encounter another narrowing, which being patiently overcome, the first joint of the finger found more room and examined uterine cervix and the external os, which is linear antero posteriorly. The neck projects about half an inch into the vagina. The lips are thin, of normal density. Withdrawing the finger and finding the smaller opening, could succeed in penetrating only about an inch. Observed a third, smallest opening in the left vaginal wall, between the ostium vaginæ and the second opening described.

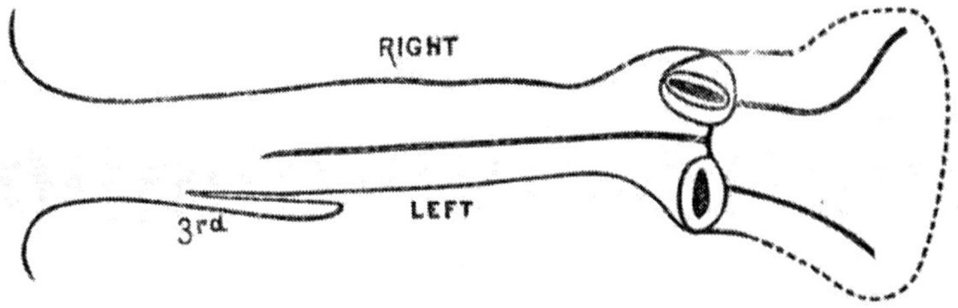

The patient would consent to no interference that could possibly cause even temporary disability for daily housework and care of an invalid mother, but agreed to return daily for a few days. After dilating without anæsthesia fifteen to twenty minutes daily for four days, could pass two fingers or a Fergusson speculum one and one-eighth inches into the right passage, and could pass one finger readily, or speculum seven-eighths of an inch in diameter into the left passage. The septum between the two passages is placed antero posteriorly. It is about an eighth of an inch thick, and has the appearance of any other portion of the vaginal wall. It begins an inch within the introitus, and extends to the uterus, making a right and left vagina of normal length. The third, smallest passage, admits a sound and extends upward an inch in the left lateral vaginal wall and ends in a blind extremity.

The right vagina discloses an uterine os three-eighths inch in length antero posteriorly, the anterior end of the slit inclined toward the median line. The sound passes readily a distance of one and three-eighths inches, entering in a direction upward and inward half that length, and then turning upward and outward. The sound moves freely in the cavity, and the lining membrane evidently contains folds. Secretion of the cervix free.

On the left side the os uteri is smaller, the opening not exceeding a quarter inch, the length being laterally. The lips are in a pouting shape, the anterior, especially, having quite a fold above it. The sound enters freely nearly an inch in a direction upward, outward and slightly backward; lining membrane apparently folded. Very little secretion. By introducing two fingers of the left hand, palm upward, the index into the right vagina and the second finger into the left, the two uterine mouths can be examined simultaneously, and this gives a very vivid impression of the condition. As to the shape of the whole uterus very little can be determined by bimanual examination, the vaginal walls being so tense and abdominal thick. By the rectum the uterus can be felt flat and wide, but no bi-lobing is apparent.

The young lady could not be persuaded to permit an examination during menstruation to determine whether the flow took place on both sides.

MEDICAL SOCIETIES—THEIR BENEFITS TO US AND OUR DUTIES TO THEM.

BY DR. WILLIAM FORSTER, RETIRING PRESIDENT VENANGO COUNTY MEDICAL SOCIETY, PENNSYLVANIA.

Though at best societies in their present form are not very old, medical associations, differing somewhat in their organization and aim, are as old as the science of medicine itself. Even in the fabulous ages it had its heroes, and some rose to the height of deification. In earlier ages those who practiced medicine were looked upon as inspired. They, in addition to belonging to a profession, constituted a class or caste. In some Asiatic nations, and among some of our Indian tribes, it is very much the same at present.

One must belong to the caste, or be able to trace his descent from it, as a necessary qualification to practice medicine.

This is the earliest form of a medical society, and though it may not possess many progressive elements, it has elements of strength.

What few investigations it did make, it kept. Its peculiar organization and position fitted it for being a good conservator; and when the star of empire took its western course, the tide of medical knowledge stored up and held sacred and secret in Asia, Egypt and Greece, flowed out and was diffused over five continents.

Hippocrates, about twenty-five hundred years ago, took the light from under a bushel. About three hundred years later the great Alexandrian school or society—for it was a society as well as a school—trimmed the light and set it higher, but it was so obscured and encompassed with exclusiveness and secrecy as to be a long time in reaching the masses.

The first societies in Germany, France and Great Britain were in connection with their institutions of learning, as they were at an earlier period in Egypt and Greece. In Rome we have reason to believe that they were more independent, as the physicians used a society seal as a label for their medicine. Truly independent society organization and work is comparatively of our own day. Even in the early part of the present century, British authority was the London, Edinburgh and Dublin colleges.

In our own country, previous to the organization of the American Medical Association, about thirty-six years ago, there was very little system in society work. That organization marks a new era in society usefulness. From it sprung the International Medical Congress, making a unit of medical investigation and progress of the world. We point with pride to Philadelphia as the city in which the association was organized, and to the able and determined stand our State has ever taken in sustaining and strengthening it. It has been a power for good to American medicine. It has elevated and is elevating the standard of our American medical colleges.

The progress in society organization, work and usefulness in the last thirty-six years is greater than in all American medical history previous to that time. We had then a few isolated independent medical societies without unity and without influence. We have at present a society in almost every county, a State society in every State, all united in an association and wielding an influence national and world wide.

Great as the benefit has been to the profession at large, it has been greater still to the individual practitioner. It has been to him a post-graduate school.

In our societies A. meets B., B., C. and C., D. They compare their investigations, experiences and theories, and each is benefited.

Our society enables us to know one another better. It is a true saying that, "no man is as good as his best deed nor as bad as his worst." Our meeting in society aids us in striking the balance and makes us more united, by forming and cementing friendships. They discourage quackery, empiricism and everything that is professionally low and mean. They encourage and stimulate purity, nobility and rectitude. They are a strength to us medically and medico-legally. All that is necessary on our part to secure us these benefits and many more which might be enumerated, is to do our duty to our county, State and national societies. I will now present to you what I believe to constitute at least part of that duty.

First. Punctuality and regularity in attendance. This increases our interest and gives the society strength.

Second. Support with our intellect. We may not all have an equal number of talents, but he that has five should use them, and he that has one should use it, and the use of that one may be just what the society needs at the time.

If we have anything we think good in theory or practice, or any interesting case, let us report to our society.

I believe everything presented should be in writing, for very few physicians are good extemporaneous speakers, and all members should have such notice of the subject of all papers to be read before the society as will give them time to prepare for intelligent discussion; for unless a man has a clear idea of his subject he is liable to wander off into a labyrinth of side issues.

When appointed for a paper, we should have it ready and be on hand to read it. We should have more papers published, and to better prepare them for publication, each society should have an editor and a publication committee, with ability and power to revise, correct and publish papers and reports of the society.

Third. We should support our society with our influence. All have an influence, and there is no neutral ground. It must be for or against.

Never was there a time when there was more need of the support of the good men in the profession. The code of medical ethics has been attacked. The American Medical association has been attacked.

An attempt has been made to make the one obnoxious and destroy the harmony and usefulness of the other.

Fourth. We should be prompt in paying our dues and all other necessary demands that may be made on us by our society. Negligence—for it is seldom or never inability—on our part may not only embarrass the society, but tend to destroy our interest in it.

I have a great regard for the Venango County Medical Society. It was the first society I joined after graduating, over twenty years ago, and I have always highly prized the friendships herein formed.

Death has taken some from us, good men and true, but I am pleased to see that we are also adding to our number so many young men, and growing in strength. Let us each do our part to keep up this growth, so that when we are weighed in the balance we may not be found wanting.

I thank you for your kind aid and forbearance throughout the year. May our society live long and prosper.

EDITORIAL.

THE LATE DR. ALFRED C. POST.

One of the old land marks of the medical profession is gone! Few men are privileged to continue in actual practice fifty-seven years! Thousands have heard him lecture, seen him operate and read his published papers. He was indeed a remarkable man. At the age of eighty he continued to operate with the freshness of youth. As a lecturer he was terse—direct to the point; as a writer he was lucid and clear; as an operator he was steady, bold and self-reliant; as a man he was a Christian.

If there was one thing more than another more prominent in his well-rounded character, it was his devotion to duty. He was a man of fine religious faith, devout in his behavior and an excellent theologian and Biblical scholar. The two things he is said to have most enjoyed were a surgical operation and a prayer meeting. He was a consistent member of the Presbyterian church, and his example of earnest, unselfish devotion to duty can not help but leave an influence for good which will last long after his brilliant surgical operations are forgotten.

Dr. Post was born in New York city in 1805, graduated from Columbia College in 1822, became a medical student in the office of Dr. Wright Post, his uncle, an eminent surgeon of a former generation. He graduated from the College of Physicians and Surgeons in 1827. After spending two years in the medical schools and hospitals of Paris, Berlin and Edinburgh, he commenced active practice of his profession in New York city, which he continued until the week before his death. He was one of the founders of the Medical Department of the University of New York, taking the chair of surgery and pathological anatomy, and at the time of his death was president of the medical faculty and emeritus professor of the clinical surgery in that institution. His funeral took place Wednesday, February 10, and the Church of the Covenant, of which Dr. Post was a member, was crowded with professional and other friends of the dead man.

ALUMNI ASSOCIATION OF THE MEDICAL DEPARTMENT OF THE WESTERN RESERVE UNIVERSITY.

The annual meeting of the Alumni Association will be held at 2 o'clock, P. M., Wednesday, March 3, in the amphitheatre of the City Hospital corner of Erie and Lake streets.

Dr. E. D. Burton of Collamer, Ohio, will be the orator of the occasion, and Prof. Proctor Thayer, the elected poet.

The president, Prof. G. C. E. Weber, will also deliver an address.

The subjects for discussion are: First, Cholera, the leading speakers being Doctors Thayer, Lowman and Kelley. Second, Diphtheria, its Aetiology and Treatment, with Dr. Knowlton of Brecksville, and Dr. Orwig of Cleveland, as leading speakers. The annual election of officers will be held, and other important business transacted.

The Hon. S. E. Williamson will deliver an address to the graduating class in the evening. The graduating exercises will be held in the First Methodist Church, corner of Euclid avenue and Erie street. There will afterwards be a reception and banquet at the Hollenden.

THE WESTERN PENNSYLVANIA MEDICAL COLLEGE.

The Western Pennsylvania Medical College has been organized and liberally endowed, and will soon assume possession of its new building on Sixth street, Pittsburgh, Pennsylvania. The course of lectures will not begin, however, until October. The faculty will be composed of the following well-known, earnest and hard-working practitioners: Professor of Anatomy, Dr. Heckelman; Professor of Physiology, Dr. Allen; Professor of the Principles of Surgery, Dr. Murdock; Professor of the Practice of Surgery, Dr. McCann; Professor of the Principles of Medicine, Dr. Shively; Professor of Clinical Medicine, Dr. Lane; Professor of Chemistry, Dr. Blank; Professor of Materia Medica, Dr. Gallagher; Professor of Obstetrics, Dr. Duff; Professor of Gynæcology, Dr. Asdale; Lecturer on Dermatology, Dr. Dunn; Lecturer on Nervous Diseases, Dr. Ayers; Lecturer on Orthopædic Surgery, Dr. King; Lecturer on Genito-Urinary Diseases, Dr. Thomas.

SOCIETY PROCEEDINGS.

PROCEEDINGS OF THE NORTHEASTERN UNION MEDICAL SOCIETY.

SIXTIETH QUARTERLY SESSION, HELD AT AKRON, OHIO, TUESDAY, FEBRUARY 2, 1886.

The president, Dr. J. E. Dougherty, in the chair.

Dr. Bauer, of the Committee on Obituaries, was instructed to prepare a fitting memorial to be read at the next meeting upon the death of Dr. J. C. Ferguson of Mogadore.

Dr. Pierson read a history of a clinical case. The clinical committee, consisting of Drs. Hitchcock, Bauer and Rowe, after examination, reported the case to be one of chronic pleuritis with adhesions and effusion, and recommended alterative treatment.

Dr. Fisher read a report of a case of puerperal convulsions, in which venesection had been resorted to with favorable results.

In the discussion which followed, Dr. Shively said he did not believe in blood-letting, but would rely upon *drastic cathartics* and anæsthetics.

Dr. Wright, in a practice of fifty years, had employed blood-letting in a few cases with good results.

Dr. Everhard had seen several cases, and favored the use of anæsthetics, but objected to the use of morphine on the ground of the supposed uræmic pathology of puerperal convulsions.

Dr. Howard thought Dr. Fisher's treatment of the case good, and believed emphatically in blood-letting, and also in the use of arterial sedatives, such as verat., vir., etc.

Dr. T. C. Miller believed in thorough narcosis, giving morphine hypodermically until the effects were noticeable on the respiration. Anæsthetics are good, but can not be given continuously. The physician giving the anæsthetic, when the convulsions cease will not crowd the anæsthetic, and almost before he is aware of it the convulsions will return. We have much to learn about the pathology of puerperal convulsions. The speaker does not believe it to be uræmic. All of his cases in which he gave narcotics thoroughly from the first recovered; cases in which he used blood-letting died.

Dr. Vance believed that the treatment advised by Dr. Miller would result disastrously in many cases, and spoke at some length, showing that the latest authorities believed the true pathology of the trouble to be uræmic.

Dr. Pixley asked, after hearing so many opinions from so many distinguished speakers: "What is Dr. Pixley going to do to-night if he meets a case of puerperal convulsions? One speaker swears, if you bleed, your patient will die; another swears, if you don't bleed, your patient will die; a third says, you must give opium; another says, you must not; another says, you must give anæsthetics; another veratrum, another cathartics." Now, after all of this light upon the subject, he would do as he always has done—apply cold to the head, warmth to the extremities, maybe give a little opium, possibly bleed a little, equalize the circulation, and deliver as soon as possible. Some of his patients will live and some will die.

Dr. Howard submitted to the society, for signatures, a petition to the State Legislature in the interests of what is known as the "Sharpe bill," for the creation of a State Board of Health and a State Board of Medical Examiners.

Adjourned to 1:30 P. M.

AFTERNOON SESSION.

On motion of Dr. Vance it was decided to hold the next meeting in Cleveland, and on motion of Dr. Scott the Cuyahoga County Medical Society was invited to meet with this society.

It was also decided that, because of the session of the American Medical Association occurring in May, the meeting of this association be held on the first Tuesday in April.

Drs. A. R. Baker and W. T. Corlett were appointed a committee on arrangements for the meeting in Cleveland.

An election of officers for the ensuing year was held, with the following result: President, Dr. J. W. Shively of Kent; first vice-president, Dr. A. C. Belden of Akron; second vice-president, Dr. T. C. Miller of Massillon; recording secretary, Dr. L. S. Ebright of Akron; corresponding secretary, Dr. A. K. Fouser of Akron; treasurer, Dr. E. W. Howard of Akron.

Dr. Dougherty at once relinquished the chair to his successor, and in so doing begged to be excused from the customary valedictory address because of his having lately given up the practice of medicine and being now very busily engaged in the duties of a county office.

Dr. Shively, the president-elect, after thanking the members for the honor conferred upon him and commending the society upon its active prosperity and scientific advancement, entered upon the duties of the office.

The recording secretary and treasurer submitted their annual reports, which, on motion, were referred to the finance committee. The committee, after making a thorough examination of the accounts of the secretary and treasurer, reported them as correct, but at the same time recommending a more accurate system of book-keeping in the future, as well as the passage of a resolution providing for an annual due from each member.

Dr. McEbright gave notice of his intention to introduce such a resolution at the next meeting.

Dr. Loughead, the appointed essayist, read an interesting paper upon the Metric System, reviewing the many advantages which might be gained by its adoption by the medical profession.

Dr. D. B. Smith read a report of a case of hysterical blindness (see page 212 of this number), and followed with a verbal report of a very peculiar case of exfoliation of the epidermis.

Remarks on the cases reported were made by Dr. Corlett and others.

Dr. Hitchcock reported a case of malpresentation, in which, by manipulation and the slight aid of forceps, delivery was accomplished with safety to both mother and child.

Dr. Corlett spoke on the method of prescribing the bromide of arsenic. He said the most trustworthy way was the alcoholic solution, which he had been in the habit of diluting it in the strength of one grain to eight ounces of simple elixirs without precipitation. Care must be taken that no water be added before the bromide of arsenic is dissolved in alcohol. Spoke favorably of its use in the class of skin diseases known as *nenrosecutanae.*

Dr. Ebright reported the case of a man who had swallowed a silver dollar. Dr. Pixley told of a similar disposition of a five franc piece, and Dr. Everhard related a recent attempt by a lady to swallow the gauge of a sewing machine. The three cases terminated favorably, though the last mentioned required the aid of a surgeon.

The chair announced the following as the standing committees for the ensuing year:

Admissions—Drs. D. B. Smith, E. Hitchcock, S. Pixley.

Publication—Drs. B. B. Brashear, T. H. Phillips, H. M. Fisher.

Finance—Drs. T. McEbright, M. M. Bauer, L. P. Proehl.

Ethics—Drs. X. C. Scott, A. M. Sherman, E. Conn.

Obituaries—Drs. W. C. Jacobs, N. S. Everhard, E. K. Nash.

The appointments for the next meeting are as follows: Essayist, Dr. A. C. Brant; alternate, Dr. W. T. Corlett. Lecturer, Dr. E. W. Howard; alternate, Dr. B. B. Loughead. Reports of cases, Drs. McEbright, Phillips, Peck, Vance and Starr. Topic for discussion: "Functions of the Cerebellum," to be opened by Dr. Brashear.

After tendering a vote of thanks to the city council for the use of the council chamber, and voting two dollars to the janitor of the building, the society adjourned to meet in Cleveland on the sixth of April.

A. K. Fouser, *Recording Secretary.*

NEW BOOKS.

'An Essay on the Pathology of the Œsophagus.' By John F. Knott. Dublin: Fannin & Co.

'The Operative Treatment of Intra-Thoracic Effusion.' By Norman Porritt, L. R. C. P., Lond., M. R. C. S., Eng. London: J. & A. Churchill.

'On the Pathology of Bronchitis, Catarrhal Pneumonia, Tubercle, and Allied Lesions of the Human Lung.' By D. J. Hamilton. London: Macmillan & Co.

We can well imagine the interest with which some practitioner in a comparatively isolated locality—in the sense of being far from some one of the great Atlantic cities where all new medical and surgical works are kept in stock—reads over the titles of forthcoming works in the particular department in which he is most concerned, and the eagerness with which he anticipates their arrival after he has gone so far as to order them. It may be, in this catarrhal land of ours, that it is throat and chest diseases he is studying, and that the above works excited his interest and drew from his pocket his hard earned dollars. If so, who can doubt that emotions of pleasure warmed his heart as he contemplated the instruction to be gained and the information to be acquired from their perusal? For who would dare write on the pathology of the œsophagus, if he had nothing to say? or descant on the operative treatment of intra-thoracic effusion, if he was not qualified by learning and experience to speak on the subject? But, lest the doubter be abroad in the land, look further to the vouchers of the title page or the preface. The first work on our list is "the Essay to which was awarded the Gold Medal of the Pathological Society at the close of the Session, 1876-77." The second, "the Essay to which the Medical Society of London awarded the Fothergillian Gold Medal, 1883." Can anything be more satisfactory? It is true that our last work boasts no such authoritative endorsement, but then as the author is a professor of pathological anatomy at Aberdeen, its other imperfections—from this standpoint—we can imagine passed by, and the book, not without misgivings, may be ultimately ordered with the rest.

What is the consequence? Two of the books will prove extremely unsatisfactory, and but one will be found to fulfill in any way the anticipations of the purchaser. The work on the œsophagus is the production of an undergraduate—a creditable performance for a student, but by no means the work any practitioner, not a friend of the writer, would care to purchase. Mr. Porritt's treatise is good to that degree that one feels aggrieved that his friends permitted him to publish anything until he had produced something first-class—for he is evidently a young man of ability. Practical surgeons who have arrived at years of maturity, not infrequently have occasion to notice that young men of brilliant parts who enter upon the practice of that art, seem to think they are unjustly kept in the background because no notice is taken of their efforts to gain position in their profession by the arts of the rhetorician or the tricks of the essayist. Nevertheless, no man can become a surgeon, save by surgical works, or be entitled to speak as one except he be a man of learning or experience—or both.

After so much that is unpleasant, it is a pleasure to turn to a work of a radically different kind. In 'Hamilton's Bronchitis,' the reader will find a treatise that is a mine of pathological lore; a work every page of which is suggestive and instructive. It possesses the rare quality of being interesting to an unusual degree, and its perusal will be a substantial pleasure to all its readers.

'The Physician Himself.' By D. W. Cathell, M. D. Fifth edition. Baltimore: Cushings & Bailey.

It is rather humiliating to the physician who is interested in equipping his brain to successfully combat disease to find himself distanced by the individual who rides into a paying practice in a fine carriage. But we must take the world as we find it, and so long as people are judged by what they seem and not by what they are, such books as the 'Physician Himself' will be demanded. What shall we eat, and where shall we sleep, and how shall we be clothed withal, are, like the poor, always with the doctor.

Dr. Cathell has succeeded quite well in showing the importance of business tact and sagacity in promoting the welfare of the physician. He gives rules as to the best methods to pursue toward patients both in the office and out, so as to line the doctor's pocket-book. He tells him how to dress, how to walk, how to sleep and how to eat, what kind of signs to display, gives hints as to the selection of an office, together with suitable furniture, etc., etc.

'Post-Mortem Examination.' By Professor Rudolph Virchow. Translated by T. P. Smith, M. D., from the fourth German edition. Philadelphia: P. Blackson, Son & Co.

In this admirable little work, Prof. Virchow gives a brief account of his early experience as Prosector in the dead-house of the Berlin Charity Hospital, and traces under his auspices the development of a systematic method of conducting post-mortem examinations. He also criticises, explains and illustrates the regulations which have been promulgated throughout Germany for the guidance of medical jurists in performing autopsies and drawing up reports.

He also gives three interesting cases in which the post-mortem examinations were performed by himself, the order of sequence enjoined by the regulations being closely adhered to. They may be taken as examples of the way in which all post-mortem examinations for medico-legal purposes should be conducted. It is much to be wished that a method similar to the one which has received the high sanction of Prof. Virchow were adopted in this country. One hundred and thirty-eight pages, neatly bound in cloth, with a number of plates. Price $1.50.

The Seventh Annual Report (1885) of the Ohio State Pharmaceutical Association contains, besides the constitution and by-laws and history of the organization, a number of interesting articles. One of them, by S. J. Nicolay, M. D., of Hamilton, Ohio, is in reply to Query No. 1—"Do the Various Fluid Extracts of Hydrastis Canadensis, Made Without Alcohol, Contain all of the Active Principles of the Drug?" The writer says that, properly, this extract "should not contain alcohol, since the alcoholic extractive essentially contains resin, which, being an irritant to inflamed mucous surfaces, is a detriment in a large majority of cases to which it is otherwise applicable." As to whether the various fluid extracts of this drug, made without alcohol, contain *all* the active principles of the crude article, he concludes, after an examination of six specimens from different manufacturers, that "each specimen was found to contain portions of the two known alkaloids—berberine and hydrastine—in their varying proportions." "As to whether these samples contained the alkaloids in as large quantities as the respective samples of the crude drug from which they were made, was not determined, but probably they did." If this is true, the fluid extract, without alcohol, will be as effective as that made with alcohol, beside being quite miscible with water for topical application, injections, etc., without becoming turbid and depositing resin.

Query 24—"*What* is the Most Effective and Pleasant Disinfectant?"—is answered by L. Sollman of Canton in an essay in which he treats: 1. "As to what is that something which disinfectants are intended to counteract." 2. "What articles are disinfectants, and what is the way in which they effect disinfection." 3. "Which of them is practically useful, and which is the most practical way of using them under various conditions."

A copy of the report can be had by forwarding fifty cents to the secretary, Lewis C. Hopp, Cleveland, O.

NOTES AND COMMENTS.

The Graubuch of the General Hospital of Vienna.—From this very interesting report for 1884 we learn the following: At the end of '83 there remained in the hospital 1,672 patients; of these 1,037 were males and 635 females. In '84, 23,937 patients were admitted, 14,801 males and 9,136 females. Discharged as cured, 12,532; improved, 4,485; uncured, 2,857. At the end of December, 1884, the number of patients remaining in the hospital was 1,742.

The maximum of sickness among males was reached in January (1,179); among females in May (740). The minimum among males in the month of August (842); among females in September (588).

It is somewhat interesting to note among the victims of pulmonary tuberculosis, the proportion furnished by various occupations. Two hundred and four day laborers, 113 shoemakers, 90 blacksmiths, 76 cabinetmakers, 71 turners, 30 coachmen, 19 butlers, 19 waiters, 8 landlords, 6 musicians, 6 servants, 4 conductors, 2 janitors, 1 stenographer, 1 chorister, 1 turnkey, etc. The proportion of deaths from tuberculosis expressed in percentage of the whole number of deaths was as follows: June, 5.6; April, 4.7; March, 4.4; August, 4.3; May, 4.2; February, 4.1; January, 3.9; October, 3.6; July, 3.2; November, 2.9; September and December, 2.8.

The most rheumatism occurred in May (84), most typhus in September (19), most bronchitis in March (210), the most pneumonitis in April (78), the most catarrh of the digestive organs in July (81).

Winter Prurigo, says Dr. Corlett in a clinical lecture, a common and most annoying disease of the skin in this climate, must be regarded as a *local neurosis.* In its treatment internal medication avails but little, excepting in severe cases where the paroxysms of itching occur several times during the four and twenty hours, when hydrobromic acid may be used with marked benefit. It is in local measures, however, that we are effectually able to control it.

At the outset of a paroxysm apply caustic potash in strength varying from x to xxx grains to the ounce of water, to which a drachm of glycerine may be added, after which the following should be added:

R - Menthol - ss.
Acidi carbolici - ss.
Sodii benzoati - ij.
Ung. aquae rosae - iij.
Cerae alba q. s. - Misce.

In mild cases, by omitting the caustic potash, the following lotions will be sufficient:

R - Menthol - j.
Alcoholis - ij.
Acidi carbolici - ss.
Sodae benzoati - j.
Aquae rosae - vj.
Misce.

Dr. G. E. Paget of Cambridge is to have a K. C. B. bestowed on him, and Dr. William Roberts of Manchester is to be knighted. Dr. Paget is Regius Professor of Physic in the University of Cambridge, and a brother of Sir James Paget, the eminent London surgeon. Dr. Wm. Roberts is Professor of Clinical Medicine in the Victoria University. In neither case can the title of "Sir" enhance the distinguished professional reputation already enjoyed by each of these gentlemen.—London Correspondence N. Y. Medical Record.

At the end of November the Curatorium of the General Polyclinic of Vienna held its first meeting according to its new constitution. President Bezecny and Vice-Presidents Dompropst, Marshall and Neumann-Spallart were unanimously reëlected. The chairman, Baron Bezecny, next greeted the new curators, and stated that the object of the meeting was to raise a large sum of money to erect a small hospital for emergency cases. Upon request of the chair, Prof. Schnitzler gave a brief report of the work of the Polyclinic from January 1 to November 25, 1885. Over thirty-two thousand patients were treated. The number of hearers, almost entirely doctors, during the semester year of '84-5, reached the height of four hundred and fifty-four. Among these were one hundred from Austria and Hungary, and almost as many out of the German empire. Then follow from other European States—Russia, England, Sweden and Norway, Belgium and Holland, Italy and Greece. America was represented by more than one hundred attendants; but also Asia, Africa and Australia furnished hearers to the Polyclinic. Prof. Schnitzler then left the subject of the report and moved that it be made the ambition of the Polyclinic to erect a Polyclinical hospital. This motion, after a very brief debate, was unanimously adopted.

On account of the death of Prof. Geo. Hunert, A. M., M. D., the chair of Theory and Practice of Medicine is vacant in the Medical Department of Wooster University in this city. As yet a successor has not been decided upon.

Third Annual Meeting of the Ohio State Sanitary Association.—We regret that the programme of this meeting, which was held in Columbus, O., Feb. 25-26, was not received in time for publication in our last number. A number of practical papers were read, some of which we shall present to our readers.

Drs. Scott, Ashmun and Herrick, of Cleveland, presented papers at the meeting of the State Sanitary Association.

Dr. J. H. Gleeson of 87 Bond street met a sudden death on the evening of February 22, at Gerling & Haber's drug store, No. 283 St. Clair street. It is reported that Mr. Haber handed him by mistake a couple of ounces of a mixture of carbolic acid and glycerine, which the doctor swallowed and expired in a few minutes. The inquest will bring out the facts.

Dr. Geo. F. Leick is in New York City, where he expects to remain several months.

Dr. A. B. Carpenter, who has been abroad in the hospitals of London and Berlin during the past year, has returned to Cleveland.

Dr. H. G. Sherman, owing to ill health, has gone south for the winter.

HOW DOES AMERICAN JOURNALISM AID THE DEVELOPMENT OF THE MEDICAL PROFESSION?

The New York Medical Journal says that "it regards the great distinctive service of American medical journalism as shown mainly in its counteracting influence in removing the pedantry shown in the medical colleges, and encouraging the expression of original thought in young men." Surely, it were a great thing to remove the stupidity engendered by medical schools, and to draw forth the powers of original thought which are dormant in the young doctor. Of the truth of this view we have no question, nor can any editor of any experience or success fail to have many personal experiences in this sort of work. In the very best sense of that term, the medical editor is a teacher; and this, too, in causing others to work for the common good. The education follows from the efforts of the young doctor to learn something of profit or interest to the profession, and then place this before the profession in the most attractive shape. The medical editor, in order to make his journal a success, is compelled to get the best work expressed in the best way. Most of the older members of the profession have never learned to write, and as they become burdened with the cares of a large business, it becomes impossible for them to learn the art of writing. Much they possess of positive value to the profession, but from the defect of not being able to write with comfort, their knowledge dies with them. The medical editor can get little help from them. There are a considerable number of the members of the medical profession who could not write a decent article, if they had any distinct ideas to put in it. Obviously, the medical editor can do nothing with this class. But there is another class of doctors, who have the general culture and the brains, but are too modest to think of writing for the benefit of their seniors. From this class the medical editor draws most of his working colaborers. By encouragement, by personal solicitation, by aid in matters of reference, by stimuli of ambition, of professional pride, by appealing to the sense of his obligations to do for the general profession that which lies in his power, many of this class are brought into active service in medical journalism. Having encouraged to habit of expression, the editor stimulates the habit of original research. Of course, different individuals will be stimulated in different directions. So, at last, the editor will have writers in every portion of the field of the art and science of medical surgery. Hence, it comes about that the editor sends men to work with the microscope, in the chemical laboratory, in the pharmaceutical laboratory, in the physiological laboratory, in the anatomical room, in the hospital, in the dispensary, in the tomes of medical literature of every language and of every age. In short, he has these men at work in every field congenial to them, and such that they can reach it.

In a very real sense, an editor is like a captain of a ship—he shows his abilities not so much in what he does himself, as in what he can get others to do. That there are not more really good medical journals, is due to the fact that there are really few medical men having the power of getting others to work in the fields leading to medical journalism.

When a young doctor has begun to realize that he can talk to the entire medical profession, life and study takes an entirely new aspect. The day of small things is past, and the day of an enlarged and enlarging manhood has come to him. One who does realize this truth will never write a poor article for publication. The poor articles come from quite a different sort of men. These the medical editor gradually weeds out.

Of this direct and indirect influence upon the conduct of medical colleges, and upon medical societies and medical publishers, writers of medical books, and the relations of medical men, we have not time to speak. But in all these things the medical journal is the means by which the process of both good and bad education goes forward. Out of all these educational processes the medical profession is slowly rising higher in its development.

To every young man who would make the most of his powers, we say: think, observe, and write for the medical press constantly. It may be that one article a year is all that any particular person can produce. It may be that longer time will be required, but whether the time be long or short, be sure to begin and keep up the habit of correct thinking, constant study and correct and frequent writing.—Detroit Lancet.

www.ingramcontent.com/pod-product-compliance
Lightning Source LLC
Chambersburg PA
CBHW071716130725
29531CB00036B/1705
9781023347440